The Solution For Back Pain Relief

How To Relieve Back Pain And Feel Better In One Week – Exercises And Best Practices. No More Back Pain!

by Erika Sanders

Medical liability disclaimer

The information contained in this book is intended as reference material only and not as medical or professional advice. The information contained herein is intended to give you the tools to make decisions about your lifestyle and health. It should not be used as a substitute for any treatment that has been prescribed or recommended by a doctor.

This material is written with the express purpose of sharing educational and scientific information, obtained from the studies and experiences of the author, professionals, health advocates, scientists, and nutritionists.

In no way is the information contained in this book intended to diagnose, prevent, treat, or cure any disease, nor is it intended to prescribe any of the techniques, materials, or concepts that are presented as a form of treatment for any diseases or medical conditions.

The author and the editor are not health professionals and expressly waive any responsibility for adverse effects that occur as a result of the suggestions or information contained herein.

The information in this book may not be compatible with conventional medicine or the opinions of some doctors. However, it is well documented and supported by many doctors, scientists, and health professionals. Before starting any practice related to health, diet, or exercise, it is highly recommended that you consult your doctor.

Introduction

From the base of the skull to the birth of the lower limbs, the spine is a support for the body trunk. Locomotor skills such as walking, jumping, crawling, spinning, pushing, and running, as well as non-locomotor skills such as twisting, swaying, bending, stretching, and bending, have an essential collaboration with this part of the body.

As with anything that physically supports a structure, in order to carry on without problems related to those locomotor and non-locomotor skills, it must be in good health. These welded bones are made up of discs and everything that converges there, such as the spinal cord, muscles, and ligaments of the back – but when they present problems and pain may appear. Eventually it can even compromise some or all locomotive and non-locomotive actions.

Most people, young or old, have suffered from back pain – the causes are often found in the spine. These pains can come from a trauma, old or recent injuries, or they may be due to natural wear and tear due to aging. Although, these pains can also develop due to a poor quality of life. A sedentary lifestyle or, at the other extreme, excessive physical activity can cause inappropriate use of the spine, as well as being overweight or consuming food lacking essential nutrients. This will invariably result in discomfort in the part of the body we are considering; discomfort which may be mild or, worse, to the point of causing disability. Continuous stress, the evil which is so common in this day and age and that one must learn to control, can produce serious disturbances in the fundamental support structure of the body.

When an area of the spine hurts constantly after a blow or collision has been suffered, or even when it hurts without knowing what the cause is, you have to consult the doctor. It is advisable to obtain an accurate diagnosis, which allows focused treatment in order to avoid later major problems.

Through these pages we propose to discuss the spine exhaustively, from both the point of view of its anatomy and the diversity of problems that can be generated in that area.

We think it is important to go into such detail because it is necessary to understand the vital functions of the spine, in order to be fully aware of the need to take care of this part of the body if we want to enjoy good health.

Now, at this point, readers may be wondering; *how can it help me to read this extensive book?* The question is very astute, as nobody has time to waste.

The truth is that, however much we abound in anatomical and functional details, our purpose is not to make known a manual anatomy of the spine. Our purpose goes much further; we want to be useful and contribute to providing natural relief to people suffering from diseases related to the spine.

In particular, what utilities are we going to provide? We will refer, in detail, to physiotherapy which is a specialty form of medicine that uses natural, mechanical elements in terms of physical exercises and movements. Physiotherapy can provide a lot of help to a person suffering with spinal problems. The important thing is that it does not use medication, which can produce unwanted side effects, or invasive procedures. Physiotherapeutic healing instead goes to the collaboration of natural agents such as water, air, electricity, light, sound, heat, and cold. It also goes to the mechanical agents of healing such as gymnastics and massages. Here we will disclose everything you can do for your own pain, including how to properly apply cold or heat and carry out simple, specific exercises.

As we said before, the first thing is to have a medical diagnosis. Then, if you are sure that the pain originates from postural problems or a poor quality of life such as excessive and continuous stress, we recommend analyzing the information we provide because we know it to be very useful.

We do not stay within theoretical considerations but give practical exercises. These are exercises that, by themselves and through consistent use, can alleviate and even eliminate pains in the area of the back.

We are in the position to affirm that we offer our readers a therapeutic program for some of the ailments related to spinal problems. We will include a wide variety of suggestions and activities to ease pain, avoid aggravating the ailments, and prevent disorders in the future.

In some cases, the ideas we offer may consist of practicing activities with an instructor in an appropriate place such as Pilates, swimming, or an aquagym. In other cases, we describe the exercises in such a way as to be able to do them correctly and regularly at home. Likewise, we will emphasize taking care of the spine in all the tasks that we carry out daily. It is incredible how, by simply changing the way we go about our daily tasks, we can alleviate the spine.

A well-informed person, when it comes to a health problem that afflicts them, will be in a better position to face their illness, administer treatment, and even fully recover. If you do have to go to the doctor, you will be in a better position to request appropriate professional support and rid yourself all doubts regarding what is best for your health. A proactive patient always receives greater advantages than a passive patient who waits for others to decide for them.

Our greatest satisfaction would be that this book about spine health is useful in providing knowledge and understanding. Consequently, our goal would be to help people suffering from pain in the back area. Thank you very much for trusting in what we have to say - and go ahead with reading!

Chapter 1 – Anatomic References

The spine is formed by a set of welded bones, which extend from the base of the skull to the birth of the lower limbs, where they join the pelvis through the sacral-iliac joint. Not only is it composed of the bony part, but it also the spinal cord, muscles, and ligaments converge there. It is an essential support structure for the body, which allows you to remain upright and at the same time flexible.

If you see an image of the spine intact and with normal features, seen from the back appears it appears to be straight. On the other hand, if you see an image of the spine in profile with normal characteristics, it appears with three important curvatures, almost like the shape of an S.

The vertebrae, short bones articulated and lubricated by synovial fluid, overlap and align. There are seven cervical vertebrae; the first is called Atlas (in the upper part of the back), then there are twelve dorsal or thoracic vertebrae (in the middle part of the back with ribs attached), and five lumbar vertebrae (in the lower part of the back). At the lower end of the column there are bones called sacrum and coccyx, formed by unarticulated vertebrae because they are fused. Five sacral vertebrae make up the sacrum and four or five coccygeal vertebrae make up the coccyx.

The vertebral column surrounds and protects the spinal cord, the part of the cerebrospinal system contained in the spinal canal, from the foramen magnum to the lumbar region. We speak of the cerebrospinal system because the cord is the brain's extension. What is the brain? Nothing less than the set of organs that are part of the nervous system, contained in the internal cavity of the skull.

As you will see, the spine is not only a support for the body but also contributes to the activity of the nervous system; the nervous system is formed by the set of nerves, ganglia, and nerve centers which ensure the coordination of vital acts and the reception of sensory stimuli.

Also, the muscles and ligaments of the back converge in the spine. The vertebrae, as well as the vertebral discs located between each vertebra, are responsible for absorbing the impact when performing locomotor and non-locomotor skills. The vertebrae act as the true protective shields of the spinal cord. The middle vertebrae are separated by intervertebral discs which engage with a facet joint. These are small joints located between and behind the adjacent vertebrae.

Chapter 2 – Causes Of Spine Problems

One or several issues can cause problems in the spine, however, the causes are sometimes difficult to establish with precision. There may be problems arising from infections, injuries, strokes, diseases of various kinds, and bone changes due to age. It may even be influenced by a genetic factor, such as ankylosing spondylitis which is a type of arthritis that affects the spine and can be inherited.

When you start to feel pain in your back it may be due to a problem that originated some time ago but had not yet manifested.

If there is trauma, it causes injury to the tissue or even bone. The trauma may have been caused by a car collision, lifting an excessive weight, or having suffered some violent impact, such as during the practice of a sport.

Sometimes the pain disappears a few days after the accident but reappears later. When the spine is observed on a radiographic plate, it may be discovered that there is a lesion, which can be in the joint cheeks, vertebral discs, or joints.

The vertebral column may be painful due to misaligned or dislocated vertebrae. The vertebral discs, which serve as cushioning, may have been displaced due to muscular imbalances, by a herniated disc, or bulging due to escape of the internal substance, a vertebral subluxation, a fracture anywhere in the spine, or, what is even more serious, a fracture combined with a dislocation. Any bone-related change that occurs in the spine can compress the marrow or nerves and, therefore, cause a lot of pain. Also, pain can be a response to various diseases. There may be facet joint disease or facet syndrome, which is when the facet joints are irritated. There may be spinal stenosis or narrowing of the spinal canal opening, or there may be spinal arthritis, which is an inflammation of the joints. There may be osteoarthritis of the spine, which is when the joints become altered and degenerate, although they do not become inflamed.

Degenerative disc disease is common in older people, although younger people can suffer from osteoarthritis or rheumatoid arthritis, which causes degeneration in the vertebrae. There may be a spondylolysis or an isthmic spondylolisthesis, which is what is known as a herniated disc - when part or all of a vertebra moves to another vertebra.

There is also coccydynia, which affects the coccyx or what we commonly call a sweet bone, and there may even be aranoiditis, which is an incurable inflammation that occurs in the arachnoid lining of the brain and spinal cord.

All the causes that we have just mentioned are physical. However, there are emotional causes that can affect the health of the spine. What is the main type of emotion that can affect the health of the spine? Continuous stress or situations where the body and / or the mind is required to perform above normal, which ends up negatively affecting us emotionally and organically.

Specifically, stress can cause tension myositis syndrome which originates in the mind due to some repression and ends up cause an intense pain in the spine. It is commonly referred to as back pain related to stress. Also, a person suffering from depression adopts a position that helps increase lumbar lordosis (concave curvature backwards in the lumbar vertebrae) and can cause pain in that area.

On the other hand, as people age they begin to lose the strength of their muscles, tendons, and bones. Due to a lack of lubrication, the discs become more rigid and degenerate or change their nature. The spurs or protuberances appear, which can compress the vertebral canal.

The spine also ages and loses its functionality in part. In fact, it's common to experience back pain from the fourth decade of life onwards. The lifestyle of the person will depend on how much the functionality of the column has been preserved. There are young people who are sedentary, do not take care of their position, and are of an excessive weight, so they will have lost the vitality of the column long before what the biological clock marks as old age. Other people comply with a good diet and exercise regime, developing strength and resistance in their muscles, so they will be less likely to suffer disadvantages in the health of their spine.

Even when natural aging occurs, the harmonious functioning of the nervous and muscular systems will have the best possible level of preservation.

The spine can also be affected by pregnancy, when the weight of the tummy begins to cause aching and discomfort. There are usually more problems in the spine when the woman gains too much weight, well above the kilos necessary to carry the pregnancy to term.

In this report we will repeatedly refer to lifestyle because it is essential to understand that, if you do not live in a healthy way, you cannot pretend to have a healthy spine. As it is a fundamental part of the organism and the vertebral bones, spinal cord, muscles, and ligaments that converge in the need to remain healthy. In order for this, one must have a diet with all needed nutrients - without forgetting the importance of calcium.

Healthy eating should neither have excess calories or nutritional deficiencies. Regular physical activity is as important as it is to break harmful addictions to substances such as alcohol, tobacco, or drugs. In the case of nicotine addiction, it has been proven that it decreases nutrients and can affect the health of the spine. The cough experienced by smokers can also cause severe back pain.

Chapter 3 – Obtaining a diagnosis

When the health of the spine is compromised the pain comes, an annoying feeling that can range from mild to intense. Sometimes the pain lasts for a few days - when it lasts almost a whole month it can be classified as acute pain. This type of pain is usually presented by having made an excessive effort, such as lifting a very heavy object, and usually manifests in the lower back.

Other times the pain is prolonged for a period over three months and is already considered chronic pain, which may have its origin in various causes. It can also be that the pain is intermittent or recurrent, meaning that sudden pangs of pain appear and disappear every so often.

The truth is that any pain in the spine which lasts for more than three days warrants a consultation with the doctor, especially when the pain does not improve with rest or if you have a fever.

The consultation, in the first instance, can be made to a clinical doctor or directly to a trauma specialist or orthopedic surgeon. If you have had an accident or suffer from, or have suffered from, other diseases such as cancer, you still have to delay the medical consultation. Most of the time, spinal problems have to do with lifestyle and respond to a sprain or twist, but there is a small percentage of cases where an underlying disease has to be treated. Cauda Equina Syndrome, a tumor, or a spinal infection, for example, are diseases that require urgent medical attention.

The doctor, if he does not yet have the patient's medical history, will prepare an anamnesis which is the part of the clinical examination that gathers the personal, family, and hereditary data. In the medical consultation you should expose any known diseases and past surgical procedures, as well as mentioning any and all the medicines that are being taken in any form.

In general, a blood test, or blood count, and an x-ray, or plate with x-rays of the spine, are required to make an initial diagnosis. The doctor will evaluate if it is necessary to order an x-ray of the entire spine or only the part where the pain is expressed. The x-ray will expose the bones of the spine and it is very possible, with scope, to observe the problem.

The doctor can also explore postural problems and inspect the spine through touch-to-detect asymmetries, muscle atrophies, and muscle contractures, which are an expression of the problem that manifests itself.

If other studies are required in addition to the radiography, then a computerized axial tomography and/or magnetic resonance imaging may be requested. With this last study you can better observe the soft parts, such as the muscles, tendons, and tissue surrounding the spine. In very specific cases a study called a mileogram may be required, which uses a contrast substance at the same time as a computed tomography to evaluate the spinal cord, nerve roots, and surrounding tissues.

It is not always easy to obtain an accurate diagnosis. Regardless, you must follow medical indications because the pain does not simply go away after the consultation. If the doctor recommends heat and/or cold compresses, as well as exercises or even physiotherapy sessions, you must be obedient.

You may be prescribed analgesics or muscle relaxants, over-the-counter or not. Once the examinations are completed, other treatments such as steroid injections may also be available. Although evolution is a slow process, in very few cases is surgical intervention the only option.

They may also recommend the use of orthopedic devices such as a corset, hyperextension girdle, lifting belt, support harness, belts (trochanter, sacroiliac), or a molded jacket.

The point is, that it is essential to consult the doctor when the pain in the spine persists for more than three days or when there was an injury. Do not forget that there are problems in the spine that, if left untreated, tend to worsen or, in some cases, generate physical disabilities ranging from mild to severe.

Chapter 4 – First of all, prevention

If you have never suffered from pain in the area of the spine, you should prevent it from ever occurring. If you have already suffered pain in the area of the spine but it then disappeared, it is advisable to prevent it from happening again. If you are going through a problem related to the spine, some preventive measures will be useful to calm the pain and prevent further deterioration. The truth is that any measure which prevents spinal problems will also be slowing the aging process.

The action of prevention is taken to avoid any inconveniences. In this case, the aim is to avoid problems in the function of the spine and its surrounding area of the back. First of all, when we talk about taking preventive measures to keep the spine healthy, we are talking about taking preventive measures for the health of the whole of the body and the mind. Each person is a physical and psychic whole, so they must be considered as such.

Many of the problems that affect the health of the spine originate from being overweight. When a person is well above the recommended weight according to their sex and height, it overloads all the support of their torso.

Therefore, one of the essential preventative measures if you want to preserve the health of the spine is maintaining an adequate body weight, which is achieved with a balanced diet which is healthy, low in fat, and without excess of caloric foods. This should be complemented by the practice of regular, constant, low or null impact physical activity. Do not forget that obesity and the sedentary lifestyle are the first triggers of back pain. At the opposite end of the spectrum, but still tied with poor eating habits, a person will have problems with his spine when he is well below the recommended weight according to their sex and height. Such is the case of anorexia. If there is a lack of nutrients in the body then the bones, cartilage, and muscles do not receive sufficient nutrition and begin to weaken. The spine, which is mainly comprised of bone, does not maintain its strength to support the torso and fulfill its functions. It can even produce decalcification or bone demineralization which would first cause osteopenia and later osteoporosis.

On the other hand, women going through menopause, as well as the elderly, are also prone to calcium deficiency with the consequent appearance of osteopenia followed by osteoporosis. This greatly affects the spine and, if not treated as it should be, can cause serious functional problems due to the loss of strength, flexibility, and agility. You can even cause fractures due to progressive bone weakening. The fundamental preventive measures to avoid osteopenia and osteoporosis would be to maintain adequate levels of calcium, both with food (especially with the contribution of vitamins A and D) and with physical activity, which helps strengthen the muscles and tendons of the back.

Now, back pain is usually common in young people. What's going on? If we talk about prevention of problems in the spine, the first thing that can be done in everyday life is to sit, lie down, and walk properly. That is, to practice with correctness the three habitual poses that accompany any human being during the course of their life. Whether sitting in an office chair or car seat, you have to keep your back, neck, and head upright with proper support of the lumbar vertebrae.

When sleeping it is necessary to use a high-density mattress and it is preferential to do so on your side, with the legs somewhat bent. When you wake up after a good night's sleep, you should do it softly and stretch your arms, legs, and torso slightly. When you move or stands up, you must hold your spine correctly aligned so that the weight is distributed proportionally over the support of your legs and feet. (We will give more practical details on this point in Chapter X. *Caring for the Vertebral Column in Daily Life*).

Another way to prevent health problems in the spine is to avoid bad movements and overloading yourself. Do not adopt a rigid posture or make sudden movements. Neither should you lift excessive weights. If you have to move a heavy object, you have to figure out how to do so without forcing the column. There are those who place the objects above a carpet and then drag the carpet; an ingenious measure that should be seen in all cases if it relieves the overload. It is also preferable to push rather than drag. Perhaps the best thing is to ask for help, as the joint forces of two or more people will be the best relief to move the heavy object and to relax the spine by simply sharing the effort.

Chapter 5 – When the pain is installed, treatment

When the area of the spine begins to hurt, it often tends to need rest. If the pain is very intense, the gymnastic or sporting practice which is being done will be left abandone. Then there are those who remain lying down or in absolute rest, waiting for the pain to disappear. It may be that the pain is relieved without treatment, although it may also remain and even worsen.

At first it is good to rest, but at the same time there are other actions to calm the pain, such as cold and/or hot compress applications. Cold compresses may consist of applying ice wrapped in a cloth. They are usually applied to reduce inflammation when the pain is severe within the first two days.

You can then apply the hot compresses, which is either a bag with hot water or a heating pad. There are those who calm the pain with the jet of a hot shower on the affected area. Or warm a towel with the iron, roll it up, and place it on your lower back while you are sitting.

If the pain does not subside you have to consult the doctor. Also, it is not advisable to continue in absolute rest after two days because it could have an adverse effect on mobility.

If the gymnastic or sporting practice that was being carried out was very demanding with many displacements, weightlifting, and a variety of combination of intense movements, it will be necessary to abandon this practice and choose another, more passive physical activity. It is necessary to prefer zero impact activities, where the feet remain supported on the floor, or at least those that are of low impact, such as walking or gymnastics which consist mainly of stretching.

If the physical activity is completely abandoned, the muscles will tense up and will contribute to further deterioration of the health of the spine. It is necessary to continue mobilizing the joints and working the muscular resistance, albeit in a light and controlled way. (See Chapter VIII. *Some Exercises To Practice at Home*). There are oral analgesics and topical analgesics, such as ointments, to apply to the painful area. There are also non-steroidal anti-inflammatory drugs (NSAIDs) to reduce pain and swelling. We recommend reducing pain without taking medications whenever possible.

If the doctor prescribe them as part of the treatment, they should be taken directly as recommended. Medications to reduce inflammation and thereby relieve pain can negatively affect another part of the body, such as the gastrointestinal tract.

In many cases the pains diminishes through the consistency of applying cold and/or heat to distend the muscles, tendons, and ligaments. The cold contracts the muscles, deflates swelling, and numbs the pain, while the heat dilates, reduces spasms, and eases pain. Ice or a heating pad can be applied as indicated.

Do not delay in making the appropriate behavioral changes, such as improving resting and active posture, as well as not lifting or dragging heavy objects. (See Chapter VII. *What Can You Do At Home To Control Stress And So Relieve Pain?* And Chapter X. *Caring for the Vertebral Column in Daily Life).*

In summary, when the health of the spine is poor and causes persistent pain you have to consult the doctor and follow their instructions.

Basically, treatments usually consist of:

- Application of cold compresses and/or heat compresses (consult the doctor when they are convenient and when they aren ´t).
- Changes in body behavior (static and dynamic).
- Adequate exercise, especially stretching.
- Analgesics administered orally or topically to the painful area.
- Medications directed to the painful area.
- Other unconventional resources:

acupuncture, electro-acupuncture, acupressure, neuromuscular and deep tissue massage, transcutaneous electrical nerve stimulation (with electrodes), spinal traction therapy, spinal decompression therapy, and hypnosis therapy.

You should exhaust all available resources before undergoing a surgical procedure. Even a herniated discs can improve without the need for surgery, using procedures which are not invasive.

Chapter 6 – Physiotherapy, bio-psycho-social knowledge of the person

We are going to refer to a very important resource in the prevention, treatment, cure, and recovery of the health of the spine: physiotherapy. It is a therapeutic science which mainly uses natural agents such as water, sound, heat, cold, and electric pulsations. Under no circumstances does it use medicines or chemical remedies.

Although manual therapy is usually the main tool of the physiotherapist, by means of massages or similar procedures, it also usually resorts to therapy with the use of elements, such as magnetotherapy, hydrotherapy, electrotherapy, and ultrasonotherapy.

Manual massages are still a good method to relieve the irritated area, especially when there is no inflammation. They increase blood circulation, relax musculature and activate endorphins.

There are different types of massage recommended for back pain, although not all types of massage are usually performed by a physiotherapist. Some examples are neuromuscular massages, myofascial, Swiss, deep tissue, and shiatsu.

A good physiotherapist begins by asking the patient by asking them about their way of life, the way they work, if they are sitting a long time, if they are standing a long time, if they have to lift heavy objects, and if they spend many hours in front of the Computer screen or practicing activities which cause tension, such as driving a vehicle or heavy machine.

They will want to know about the physical activity you do and the time you spend doing it. It is important for a physiotherapist to view the person as a whole, with the ailments existing at the time of the consultation considered alongside the ways of acting and moving in the everyday. An individual's method of interrelating with the surrounding world is also taking into consideration. The person is thought of as a bio-psycho-social being and, in this integral sense, it must be treated in a natural way so that it can be restored.

The physiotherapist can also observe the studies that the patient approaches, such as x-rays and others. They will explore the postural problems, how the person stands, walks, sits, bends, and rotates their torso. Based on radiographic studies and areas of pain, you can perform massages and apply procedures such as magnetotherapy or localized heat. There are specialists in physiotherapy who also work with osteopathy, a type of alternative medicine that focuses on recovering the body's balance with different techniques such as energy and stretching.

Joint osteopathy focuses on working on the spine to relieve pain and restore its functions. As in the case of physiotherapy, osteopathy is considered as a holistic medicine because it considers the person in its total integration. In the same line, focused manipulation of the spine is the work of chiropractors, who use physical therapy techniques to align that part of the body. Chiropractic medicine does not focus only on symptoms but seeks the basis of the problem, without using medications or invasive healing methods.

Whether it's a specialist in osteopathy or a chiropractic specialist, you have to go to those who are known to be enrolled. Although they are alternative medicines that do not report side effects, attending a suitable one will avoid, above all, wasting time without getting results to calm the pain.

Nowadays, doctors specialized in traumatology usually refer to physiotherapy sessions once they have evaluated the patient and conducted the corresponding examinations. Physical therapy does not usually solve the problem with just one consultation. You often have to attend several sessions of therapy or the therapies that are indicated for each case, two or three times a week or as specified.

In addition to the therapeutic work in the sessions there are usually recommended exercises to perform at home. The pain tends to subside progressively, if the treatment is well-aimed at the problem and the recommendations are strictly followed.

Chapter 7 – What can be done at home to control stress and thus relieve pain?

You could say that we live in the age of stress and you can rarely escape from your condition. Work is very demanding and competitive, you live running from one task to the other and never reach the time or the money, you have contracted too many obligations and you do not know how to handle it, and the daily problems of life are beyond your capacity to solve them.

In short, you live immersed in a rhythm of life that demands and passes bill for everything. It seems that you can never slow down to think that there is no sense in the excessive demand which is imposed on the body and the mind. Actually, it does not make sense to live with such emotional overload.

But let's be more specific, what can be done at home to relieve back pain? The first thing that can be done is to stop to think about what happens to us. If you have already attended the medical consultation, while you follow the instructions you have to start working on yourself.

If you are going through a situation of continuous stress, which may have resulted in stabbing pain and other symptoms, the first thing that should be done is to relieve the body and mind of so much accumulated tension.

Perhaps the stressful situation is related to the work environment and it is difficult to resolve. You have to find a solution so that the work does not have disturb your emotions to the point of getting sick.

While possible solutions are reasoned, perhaps talking to someone close to your heart can help by providing a more objective opinion. You can start by making the home a space for relaxation and good living. Although there are also household worries, such as paying bills every month and dealing with children so that they are content in all aspects, we must think that the home is the space that depends exclusively on its owners. You have to talk within the couple, if you have one, or talk to the people with whom you live who are responsible for helping. Between you all, draw up a plan for a better life.

What can be done to live better and help relieve pain? In principle, plan the daily meals in such a way that they are suitable for all the members of the family. If the person who is going through the problem with their spine is away from home and returns in the night, dinner should be the time to eat healthily, in a relaxed and calm climate of harmony. The food in the home should be a moment of pleasure.

You also have to put the emphasis on eating healthily. It may be necessary to plan purchases and have a written daily menu, which provides balanced meals with all the necessary nutrients. Eating healthily while in a relaxed space will be two important actions to overcome back pain. Eating well will help maintain the proper body weight and provide the necessary nutrients, while eating in a climate of harmony will help reduce stress.

If you are dealing with a person who lives alone, you should not stop making food your space for relaxation and pleasure. You should think about eating healthily so it will be convenient to your daily schedule, meaning you do not lack food or overeat. You must take the time to eat. If, at midday, your work rhythm does not allow you to eat properly, at night you have to eat healthy and pleasant food that you want to taste, sitting comfortably in front of the table, listening to the music you like most or watching a television program to relax.

The time you spend at home should serve for relaxation and doing things which gratify you. We must ensure that the home is a space for the encounter with oneself. You have to plan some relaxing and motivating activity; it helps to relax the muscles, but also eases the mind of its worries.

You can listen to your favorite music, try to calm the spirit through deep breaths, and lead the mind to think about comforting things. It may be convenient to seek external help to control stress, in which case you can opt for Cognitive Behavioral Therapy (CBT) or other forms of psychotherapy. At this point we must say that it is essential to continue reading the next chapters of this book. (VIII. *Some Exercises to Practice at Home*, IX. *Gymnastics and Convenient Sports*, X. *Caring for the Vertebral Column in Daily Life*, XI. *Phytotherapeutic Help*).

Chapter 8 – Some exercises to practice at home

The following exercises to perform at home are very simple and do not have great demands. Particularly in cases of chronic pain in the area of the spine, you must perform low or no impact exercises which help strengthen muscle groups, including stretching and deep breathing.

If you are receiving medical treatment, it is recommended to consult your specialist about the execution of the exercises that we detail below.

Exercises to relax the neck or the entire spine

When we refer to the anatomy of the spine we say that it extends from the base of the skull to the birth of the lower limbs. The neck, as the first segment of the spine, is very important to keep it free of contractures.

These exercises can be done at any time of

the day, though it is advisable to make it a habit if you want to eliminate neck tension. You can schedule your exercise twice a day; in the morning when you get up and at night before going to sleep.

Sit on the floor in the position of the Buddha, with the back straight and the neck and head in alignment. Place your hands on your knees. This can also be done standing up, always taking care that the spine remains well aligned. Close your eyes and let your head fall gently forwards and then backwards, for five consecutive times.

By bringing the head back, without force, the muscles of the face should be kept relaxed and the lips loose. The rest of the body, from the torso downwards, will remain motionless during all exercises. The shoulders should also not observe any movement, although free of tension.

Next, bring the head to the right shoulder and return to the center, always in a soft way. Bring the head to the left shoulder and return to the center. Repeat the movements five times.

When the head is pulled to the side the muscles contract, just as when the head returns to the center the muscles relax.

Bring the neck forward as much as possible and return it to the center, keeping the chin focused forward. Repeat the movement five times. The back of the neck will tense and then relax.

Next, tilt your head forward, letting it fall by its own weight. Then start to turn your head slowly, five times to the right and five times to the left.

Once the described movements are finished, you have to give a pat on the neck with the back of the hands, under the chin, and on both sides.

Balance to flex the spine

Tap the back of the neck with the palms of the hands and the tips of the fingers.

Then, always in the position of a buddha with an aligned back, inhale deeply and slowly through the nose and into the lungs until you feel the abdomen expand. Meanwhile raise the arms, the hands above the head, and stretch as much as possible. Hold your hands the air for a second while first stretching to one side and then to the other.

Exhale gently through the nose until the expulsion of all carbon dioxide, while lowering the arms. You can mentally count to five when you take the air, again to five when you hold it and, finally, count to five while exhaling. Perform five consecutive deep breaths by stretching the arms upwards, which will greatly relax the area of the spine.

Sit in a seat with no back and the spine straight. Interlace the fingers of the hands and hold them around the nape of the neck. Breathe deeply and, with your hands always clasped behind your head, push your elbows back. Release the breath while closing your elbows, bringing your head down and bending your back. Stay in that position for a few seconds. Repeat the exercise five times. Practiced once a day, you will both stretch and relax the spine.

This exercise is designed to make the column more flexible and resilient. Sit on a mat with your legs and your spine straight. Put your head down. Raise both knees, leaving the feet resting on the floor. Put your hands under the knee joint, bending your spine a little.

Adopted the position described and begin the swing, taking deep air when going backwards and releasing the air until exhausted when going forward, keeping the back curved. As you move forward, both feet should rest on the ground. You have to start with short rounds until you find the maximum point of return so as not to fall. Once security is acquired in the rhythm of the swing, the legs can be extended while going backwards and bent upon return.

It would become a movement similar to that of rocking chairs, which acquire a smooth, stable, and continuous rhythm. While it seems a simple exercise, when practiced about ten times a day it brings an incredible vitality to the spine. In addition to providing a massage to the vertebrae, it is a stimulus for the current of nerve energy that runs through the spinal cord, which improves communication between the central nervous system and the body in general.

Elevation of legs and abdominal contraction

Lie on a mat on your back, with your legs extended together and arms extended to the side of your body. You have to feel that the spine is fully supported.

Contract the abdomen and inhale deeply while raising a leg to form a ninety-degree angle with the torso. Hold the air while holding the raised leg and without flexing. Begin to lower the leg slowly, while exhaling air and relaxing the abdomen.

Repeat the movement with the opposite leg. Then perform the lift with both legs simultaneously - without taking off the waist of the floor - inhaling when the legs rise without flexing and with the abdomen contracted. Exhale while both legs lower without flexing and the abdomen relaxes. Repeat five elevations with each leg and five elevations with both legs together, always in a slow manner and paying attention to the abdominal contraction.

Swim simulation on the floor or with the Swiss ball

Place yourself on a mat facing down, with your arms extended forward and your legs separated by the width of your hips. Take a deep breath and raise the left arm and right leg as much as possible without flexing.

Lower the left arm and the right leg while releasing the air. Take a deep breath again and raise the right arm and left leg as much as possible without flexing. Lower the right arm and the left leg while releasing the air.

This exercise should be done slowly but continuously, until completing five elevations on each side (alternately). It is important to accompany the exercise with deep breathing in order to better relax the spine and the surrounding area.

It is an exercise considered very important for the spine because it focuses strength on the abdomen. Strengthening the abdominal muscles helps improve body posture, both when sitting and when standing.

The simulation of swimming can also be done on a Swiss ball, which is a very useful elastic sphere because it reduces the possibility of injuring the back. We must support the belly with the ball and extend the body, arms, and legs. You must control your posture to maintain balance and not fall. Take a deep breath and raise the left arm and right leg, without flexing and as much as possible. Lower the left arm and the right leg, while releasing the air. Take a deep breath again and raise the right arm and left leg as far as possible without flexing. Lower the right arm and the left leg while releasing the air.

The Swiss ball is very suitable for relaxing the spine. Some forms of relaxation include kneeling and hugging the ball, or leaning your back on the ball and swinging slightly to massage the spine.

Elevation of the pelvis

Lie on your back with your legs elevated in flexion and the soles of your feet resting on the floor. The arms remain at both sides. Take a deep breath and elevate the buttocks while contracting with the abdomen. Release the air and remain a few seconds with the pelvis elevated, breathing harmoniously.

The head and the upper part of the back, as well as the soles of the feet, remain supported. Lower the pelvis, rest a few seconds, and repeat the pelvic elevation, always slowly, until reaching five times. This exercise is very good to perform once a day because focusing the strength in the abdominal area thereby strengthens the muscles of the back.

In fact, it strengthens the muscle group called multifidus, which is located next to the vertebrae, as well as the transverse muscle of the abdomen, which is what gives stability to the spine.

Sit on the floor with a straight spine and

legs outstretched. Cross the left foot over the right knee, supporting the planted foot on the ground. Twist the right arm around the waist. The left arm rests on the ground.

Take a deep breath and, while exhaling, bring the head, shoulders, and back rotating to the right. The leg crosses to one side and the torso rotates to the opposite side. Maintain the posture for ten seconds. While exhaling return to the starting position. Rest a few seconds and then twist with the opposite side.

This twisting movement strengthens the deeper muscles of the back and the external oblique muscle of the abdomen while aiding flexibility. Ideally, practice it at least once a day.

Chapter 9 – Gymnastics and convenient sports

We recommend, for those who are able, to adopt a style of gymnastics or sports activity that they enjoy and helps them maintain the health of the spine.

The exercises to do at home that we provided in the previous chapter are very good and produce excellent results if they are carried out daily. However, an activity practised systematically two or three times a week will be even more favorable for the problems that we address.

Hikes and stretches

If you do not have the opportunity of attending a gym, you can go on hikes on your own three or four times a week for at least thirty minutes. These involve five minutes of stretching and breathing exercises, twenty minutes of moderate walking, and another five minutes of stretching and breathing exercises.

You have to perform at least twenty minutes of

moderate walking to favor the cardiorespiratory system. The walks are part of the low impact exercises that help improve posture and provide flexibility, which are very convenient to relieve pain in the area of the spine. Care must be taken to perform them on surfaces which are not hard, such as asphalt or cement, so that the tread does not produce an impact and the joints rest.

At the beginning and end of each walk you have to stretch the muscles of the legs - especially the quadriceps. The best thing to maintain balance while stretching is to support one hand on an object that stays fixed (such as a tree, if outdoors) and with the other hand take the foot from the instep or ankle and pull it backward.

Press the foot against the gluteus, keeping the back straight and taking air through the nose and exhaling through the mouth in a deep manner.

Stay in this pose for two minutes and repeat the stretch with the opposite leg.

Next, place a stretched leg on a bench or other support.

Take a deep breath and try to touch the ankle with both hands or, if possible, the tip of the toes.

Upon reaching the maximum stretch, release the air. Keep stretching the arms and legs for a few seconds; you have to feel that the spine is stretched to the maximum. Repeat with the other leg.

With your back always straight, take a deep breath and bring one leg forward. The leg which is left behind should remain stretched without flexing.

The knee which is flexed must not pass the tip of the toes. The effort is in stretching the leg that is left behind. Release the air.

Remain briefly in this position, breathing harmoniously. Repeat the exercise with the opposite leg.

The walks, as well as the accompanying

stretches, will be a great relief for the spine. You can also choose other aerobic activities, as long as they are of low impact, such as riding a bicycle (mobile or fixed).

On the other hand, it is possible to opt for non-aerobic activities which are no impact or low impact. In activities with no impact or no impact, the feet always remain supported on the ground. The movements consist of knee bends, arm movements, hip work, and body weight transfer.

Low-impact activities also do not have jumps as at least one foot remains supported on the ground. There are very advisable activities for the subject that concerns us because they focus the strength on the abdomen, as well as repeated movements of the arms and legs, although never abrupt.

There are variants of null and low impact activities that do not attack the spine while mobilizing all joints, increasing agility and flexibility. In general, they are recommended in order to maintain strong bones and to counteract diseases such as osteoarthritis, which decreases joint mobility, and osteoporosis, which weakens bones by demineralization and decalcification. It also increases the muscular capacity to take oxygen from the blood and use it as energy, favoring the cardiovascular system. Let's list some favorable activities for the health of the spine which can be added to walks outdoors or on the treadmill, as well as to the outdoor or stationary bicycle.

We recommend that, if you are under medical treatment for spinal problems or with very intense pains, you consult your doctor to know if it is convenient to start practicing some of the activities that we will describe. It is even necessary to take the precautions in choosing physical education instructors to ensure they are suitable for the task they perform. Ultimately, the responsibility falls on the person who wants to recover and maintain the health of their vertebral column.

Pilates reformer

This activity is excellent for the health of the spine for several reasons; it focuses strength on the abdomen and thereby helps correct body posture, increases strength and muscular endurance, gives flexibility, relieves muscle tension, and improves the blood system and the lymphatic system. It is said that Pilates puts endorphins to work and thereby generates a positive mood.

Pilates *Reformer* is done using a type of mobile stretchers with springs to increase or decrease the intensity of work.

In addition, a series of elements are incorporated, such as Swiss balls, elastic bands, weights, dumbbells, canes, ropes, and drawers.

The classes are incredibly personalized because a stretcher is required for each assistant, so there is usually no more than five people under the supervision of an instructor. They usually last fifty minutes and end with a back massage, performed with the sliding of rubber balls.

It is ideal to take two or three weekly classes. If it is done in a systematic way then, after a month or so, there should already be relief in the entire area of the back. By centering the strength in the abdomen, this method contributes to strengthening and to relaxing the musculature of the back.

Hatha Yoga

Yoga is one of the preferred activities to relieve spinal problems. If you have a diagnosis that reveals a specific problem in the spine then you should consult the yoga instructor because there are postures or asanas that it are not convenient to perform.

If they work with responsibility then, in the first class, the instructor is informed about the health problems that the students may have.

Yoga exercises the body while increasing mental capacity. Through correct breathing, as well as concentration and relaxation exercises, all physical and mental wellbeing improves.

When walking, sitting, or practicing the different exercises, we must try to keep the spine erect. That is, the head, neck, and trunk must be perfectly aligned.

What happens when the spine is not perfectly aligned? The free flow of life force or "prana" is impeded. Precisely, this discipline gives a fundamental importance to the breathing and to the correct postures.

What is called Hatha yoga is the yoga of physical wellbeing, which consists of several stages of learning. For the purpose of improving and maintaining spine health, it is not necessary to advance through the higher stages of learning. There are even those who learn through a video and practice it at home.

However, if you have the opportunity of being assisted by a yoga instructor it will be much better to be able to learn to perform the different postures with correction, as well as to incorporate deep breathing, concentration, and meditation exercises.

Aquagym or aquatic gymnastics

Gymnastics in the water is ideal for spinal problems because, if you work muscle strength and flexibility, it does not cause impact through the action in water. It's even a type of gym which is recommended for people who are overweight. The water facilitates the accomplishment of the exercises, helps to stretch the muscles and relax the back, and provokes a pleasant sensation worthy of enjoying. To perform this activity, it is not necessary to know how to swim.

There are those who indicate swimming as a method to correct postural problems. However, it must be considered that not all swimming styles are recommended. For example, the butterfly or breaststroke style is not recommended.

It is also not recommended to swim in the crawl style by turning your head with each stroke, because you could be demanding too much effort from the neck. The crawl style is suitable for the spine if the head is kept under water for at least three or four strokes and, in addition, if the arms are not fully stretched but are kept flexed with each stroke.

If you want to practice swimming to improve the health of the spine then consult with your doctor and ensure you have a good instructor, who helps acquire an adequate technique for the problem that you want to correct.

Chapter 10 – Caring for the spine in everyday life

When the health of the spine has suffered due to the lifestyle that is being lives, it is obvious that the best treatment that can be faced is to change what needs to change to have a healthy lifestyle. If the problems in the spine are due to weight or stress, you have to start eating in a convenient way and performing regular physical activities. It is important to choose activities that achieve the relaxation needed by the body and mind.

We are now going to refer to attitudes rather than activities. What we propose is to review how we move throughout the day and how we rest. If something we are doing may harm the spine, we will see that it does not cost much to change it while the reward is huge. Let us examine our habitual bodily postures, whether they be static, in resting position, or dynamic/ moving.

Let's stand in front of a full-length mirror. In profile, how does our figure look? Are the shoulders and belly pushed forward? Does the head remain a little down, as if to look for

something on the floor?
Does the back bend in an exaggerated way at its
high part? Are the legs warped? Needless to say,
we are witnessing the things to forever cut from
our lives.

What would be the correct way to stand, then?
The body should be aligned from head to toe.
With regard to the feet, they should be well
supported on the ground as a comfortable
support base.

The knees should remain without flexing. The
shoulders should stand erect in line with the
hips, not tending to curl forward. The head
should be in a straight alignment with the spine,
with the chin parallel to the floor and the eyes to
the front.

The abdomen should contract a little, to help
support the body. The mirror has to return the
image of a person who is safe and at the same
time relaxed, well planted, and looking straight
ahead.

If we have a job that requires us to stand for
several hours, we have to adopt the correct
posture that we have just described. What we

can do to rest a little is the body weight from one foot to the other, alternating.

As much as possible, every hour or hour and a half we should sit down for even a couple of minutes to better rest the lower area of the spine.

With that same correct posture that we adopt standing, let's try to move. When we walk, we alternately move our legs and swing our arms a little. Despite continuous movement, the spine should remain erect, with the head aligned, the eyes forward, and the shoulders back.

You have to walk with your abdomen slightly contracted to help maintain the correct position of the spine. Here comes a very important observation; if we are going to walk for ten minutes or more, we should wear comfortable shoes.

The heels must be wide and not exceed four or five centimeters. The front should accommodate the feet comfortably. The buttress must be firm, so that the foot does not deviate or twist.

The use of templates is recommended to

promote the health of the spine, provided they are made to measure the foot.

Remain seated
Now, let's place a chair in profile in front of the mirror and proceed to sit down. The movement to sit down should be smooth until the gluteus is supported. We should never throw ourselves as if we were a bag of potatoes.

Once we have leaned on the chair, we have to proceed to rectify the pose. The buttocks must slide until touching the back of the chair; the lumbar part of the back must be perfectly supported and contained against the chair. Again, the shoulders should be opened as if you wanted to expand the chest.

The head has to be aligned to the column, with the chin parallel to the floor. The knees should be bent at right angles to the hips and both feet should rest parallel resting on the floor. The position of one leg crossed over the other is not ideal to maintain for a long time.

If we perform a job that requires many hours of sitting, it is essential to preserve the health of the column to adopt a correct working posture.

Ideally, the chair to be used should be adjustable in both height and swivel - even better with an adjustable headrest and armrest.

Both the chair and the desk or table where we work must have an ergonomic design. This is even more important in front of a computer screen.

Remember that ergonomics perform the study of biological and technological data and then apply that to the adaptation between the human being and the machine.

We must also consider the lighting, so that we do not have a distorted visual angle and we do not need to make unnecessary movements with the neck.

Beyond this, the workspace must be perfectly planned to remain seated comfortably; every hour and a half or two hours it is good to get up and walk a little.

It does not hurt to stretch your legs and arms, as well as to rotate your neck and shoulders a bit.

Lift excessive weight

Be careful with overloads. If we must lift a heavy object, we have to adopt a position that will help us with our mission. Firstly, we must place ourselves as closely as possible to the object in question.

Then separate the feet a little, which should be planted firmly and pointing a little outwards. At no time should you bend your waist or turn it.

If the object is not up to our arms, we should bend the knees and point them out (like the feet), bring the buttocks out, and take the object with both hands, always keeping the column aligned.

The load that we are going to support should not be unbalanced. Ideally, do not lift heavy objects but, if we have to do it at some time, we must take care not to damage the spine.

Position to Sleep

We have already briefly discussed how to stand and how to sit. Now we have to consider what position to adopt in sleep. First, we have to procure a hard bed - not the ones with elastics.

If we do not have a hard bed, we can fix it by placing wood between the mattress and the base of the bed. The bed should be accompanied by a good mattress of high density; it should not sink with the weight of the body. The pillow should not be too high or too low, so that the head can rest without forcing the neck.

When we have the right elements, the most convenient way to rest the spine is to sleep on its side, with slightly flexed legs (never stiff), and a placed between the legs if we are very sore.

This position relieves those who suffer from osteoarthritis or spinal stenosis. The position, with the support of the back, does not harm the spine, although the sideways position is preferred. If you fall asleep on your back, you can place a cushion under the knees and another at the lower back for comfort. On the contrary, you do not have to adopt the prone position to sleep. In that case, the column as well as the neck remain in a forced position for several hours.

Chapter11 – Phytotherapeutic Help

If you go through one of those moments when the spine seems to collapse and severe pain ensues, some herbs can be used to soothe it.

Although herbs can be useful so as to avoid the potential abuse of painkillers, there are cases in which they can replace them totally or partially. Always consult the doctor, especially if you are already taking any medication, because there could be inconvenient side-effects.

Let's see some of the herbs that can help reduce inflammation and pain in the back area.

Cayenne pepper

This spicy seasoning is known for its analgesic properties. Its components include capsaicin, a substance that, when ingested, causes a burning sensation in the mouth. By stimulating sensations, the brain reacts by producing endorphins, which work as an adequate painkiller.

In a way, it is as if the pain is deceived. Substance P transmits pain from the periphery to the brain. As substance P is neutralized, the brain does not receive pain signals from the affected area.

You can make an infusion of cayenne pepper to help reduce pain in the area of the back. Place cayenne pepper, at the size and weight of an aspirin, into a cup of boiling water. It is stirred and drunk.

In the market there are ointments and oils formulated with cayenne pepper to make topical applications. It is necessary to rub the painful area and not cover it immediately, waiting until the skin absorbs the substance.

Willow bark or willow stalk

Herbs that contain salicin (such as aspirin), which in the body becomes salicylic acid, reduce muscle pain.

It can be drunk as an infusion or decoction, adding a teaspoon of willow bark to half a liter of boiling water. Take one cup every eight hours (three cups daily). The effect is not immediate.

If you are allergic to aspirin or you are taking anticoagulants you should not use willow bark.

Ginger rhizome

This is an anti-inflammatory and analgesic. Fresh, dry or powdered, ginger has substances that deflate and reduce joint pain. You can drink two cups of ginger daily (one teaspoon per cup of water at boiling point).

You can also make an infusion and apply warm compresses on the painful area, or rub the part of the back that has discomfort with ginger oil.

Do not abuse the consumption of ginger because it could be toxic. In general, no more than two grams of ginger powder per day or no more than nine drops per day are recommended. The doses indicated can be divided into two doses.

Valerian Root

This is a grass widely used to overcome insomnia, so its use is not recommended in people who operate machinery.

It is also considered antispasmodic and a muscle relaxant. In fact, it is used to relieve muscle and joint pain.

Claw of the devil or harpagofito (plant of the hook)

This has iridoid glycosides, which acts against inflammation and pain. It is used for symptoms of osteoarthritis, low back pain, and tendonitis.

It decreases swelling, inflammation, and pain. It is obtained in extract or powder form.

Chapter 12 - in-depth study of alternative medicine

In recent years there has been an increase of people seeking to treat their diseases with alternative medicine. It is a practice that generates a great deal of controversy both inside and outside the world of traditional medicine; a subject that some experts believe does not receive enough attention.

What is alternative medicine?

The most commonly accepted definition of alternative medicine is that it is a treatment or substance which is not tested using accepted scientific standards. The most common types of alternative medicine include herbology, supplements, therapies, and activity programs that fall outside traditional medical practice and are questionable in terms of safety and efficacy. For example, acupressure massage, meditation, herbal tea, and plant extracts are popular forms of alternative medicine that many medical doctors claim to be ineffective and, in the worst case, dangerous under some conditions.

Why is alternative medicine so popular?

Alternative medicine has grown in popularity as more and more people face the inevitable pains, sufferings, and diseases that come with aging. In some cases, traditional medicine has failed to produce a cure and patients go in search of other options for the treatment of their diseases. In other cases, patients firmly believe that natural methods of treating diseases are superior to traditional medicine, so they seek treatment from alternative medicine instead of traditional medical doctors.

The risks of alternative medicine

Some of the greatest risks associated with alternative medicine come from the use of unproven, ineffective, and sometimes unsafe substances. The manufacturers of such substances often exaggerate their effectiveness or misrepresent the scientific results related to the substance. This is in order to convince consumers to buy their products, even if the use of them puts the health or wellbeing of consumers at risk.

For example, some herbal remedies are

promoted to have the ability to improve memory, speed up metabolism, or even cure diseases such as cancer or heart disease. In practice, some remedies can cause psychological damage when taken in excessive amounts, such as ephedra. Another risk is that a person with a serious condition such as cancer, heart disease, or chronic diseases will forgo more traditional treatments that have been proven effective in favor of alternative treatments which are of dubious value. They would be putting their lives at risk by treating diseases with unproven alternative medicines instead of scientifically validated traditional medicine.

Another common risk associated with alternative medicine is when a patient uses both treatment methods (traditional and alternative) but does not reveal this to their doctor. It is very common for prescribed medications to produce negative interactions when taken at the same time as alternative medicines such as herbs and plant extracts. These interactions range from decreased efficacy to intoxication, causing serious damage. If the medical doctor is not aware of any other substance that the patient is taking, they will prescribe a medication which may produce a harmful or unwanted interaction.

How to recognize potentially dangerous alternative medicines

A good rule of thumb is that if the product, substance, or therapy sounds too good to be true, it is probably dangerous. Even though you are already familiar with this cliché, it is worth repeating because it is usually true when it comes to alternative medicine. Beware of any product that claims to be "miraculous", a "scientific breakthrough", "amazingly effective", "an ancestral remedy", "a secret formula", or possesses some other attribute that supposedly makes it superior to most traditional medicine.

If you are considering an alternative form of therapy such as reflexology, acupuncture, biofeedback, or similar, carefully check the qualification of the therapy professional before undergoing treatment.

What kind of training have you received, and is that training from a reliable source? Investigate the treatment to determine if it is something that has been scientifically tested, evaluated, and found effective. Do not take the instructor's word for it and do not accept the claims of anyone who benefits in some way from referring you.

Finally, ask your doctor about any alternative medicine you are considering. If you do not feel comfortable doing so, then find another doctor with whom you feel comfortable and discuss with them the alternative medicine you plan to perform. Remember that a trained, professional doctor has the education and experience to help you make good and safe decisions about whether or not to use alternative medicine.

Alternative medicine for women's health

Since women's health is a fairly broad topic, I have chosen to focus on one aspect of women's health that continues to be a problem. There are many symptoms associated with PMS (premenstrual syndrome). Unfortunately, because each woman is different, there is no agreement about the cause or treatment of the effects of PMS within the scientific community.

What everyone agrees on is that a regular menstrual cycle is a sign of good health. However, it does not help to know that you are healthy if you have pain or mood swings which cause you to have to stay at home all day or risk having to call your best friend for bail money.

Conventional medicine can offer pills for pain, regularity, and hormone therapy, but alternatives to these forms of relief can be more comforting and have fewer side effects. While, for my part, I will not "run with the wolves", I would like to achieve a kind of balance between seeing the cramps as a "medical problem" and "a gift from Mother Earth". Give me a break, I just do not want to cry and walk around hitting people or things for a week every month!

Let's explore these options:

Acupuncture relieves pain and stress, and it can leave you feeling so relaxed that you will feel too good to want to hit someone. The same goes for massages; your masseuse can show you how to perform a self-massage on your lower abdominal region any time you need to calm your cramps. There is no medicine involved, and both alternative therapies are non-invasive.

Chinese herbal medicines are used to invent teas and poultices for the relief of PMS symptoms. These include the Kava Kava Chai tea and the Gin Seng. The most recommended teas are made of Viburnum and help with cramps, irritability, and swelling. Dandelions help with inflamed breasts, muscle spasms, and acne. Your herbalist can recommend the right combination for your individual symptoms, as well as baths and foot massages.

Osteopathy is an alternative medicine that can help with diseases of the internal organs and fight against osteoporosis. The Women's Health Center at Oklahoma State University (founded by the Osteopathic Society) sponsors the "Take Over" program, which promotes health education and alternative therapies forums for women across the country.

The Chakras and healing crystal energies are used in a variety of ways to increase blood flow (ironically, if you think about it) which decreases headaches and tension symptoms caused by PMS. This seems to work, but I prefer yoga and herbal teas - pragmatic and to the point.

Although they are not considered an alternative therapy, exercise is a great way to relieve symptoms and reduce fatigue. One form of exercise that can be considered as alternative is yoga. Gentle stretching movements and low cardiac impact are very good for menstrual symptoms.

Hypnosis is rapidly becoming the alternative medicine chosen by those with PMS. Hypnosis is oriented towards the search for causes and conditions of symptoms, to alleviate pain holistically, and eliminate the root causes of irritability and stress.

While it is obviously hormonal in nature, changes in mood due to PMS can be controlled with light hypnosis which focuses on teaching the patient that these changes are temporary, rather than taking them to heart. Now, I do not know about you, but I'm more believing of a hypnotist when they say, "it's going to be okay, it's going to get better, it's temporary" than when my husband says, "are you on your period? Ah, that explains it."

Alternative treatments for male health

There are many methods of treatment in the world today, and many are directed at men

specifically. For men, you want to make sure
you are using the best alternative method. There
are three great alternative methods that work
well on men and only men.

Herbs for men

Herbs can be used on men for different
purposes, such as the treatment of the prostate,
the male reproductive system, or for infertility.
There are many different herbs that can treat
and help these male problems; there is a specific
male herbal program that can help with all these
problems. The program includes relaxing herbs,
aphrodisiacs, testosterone enhancers,
circulatory system stimulants, and adaptogens.
These types of herbs, used regularly, can cure
the problems that men encounter every day.

Chinese medicine for men

Acupuncture is the largest and most popular of
all Chinese medicines today. Acupuncture is
being used all over the world more and more
with each passing year. Many men prefer
acupuncture to all other alternative medical
treatments. This form of Chinese medicine was
created to treat all types of diseases and

problems and has amazing results in any area. This is an art of liberation and there are many people in the world who need a liberation of some kind. Acupuncture is the way they have chosen and it works! It is one of the strongest forms of alternative medical treatment.

Yoga for men

Yoga is not just a treatment for women, men can be part of this incredible therapy of sanitation and liberation. It is a great treatment for stress and the release of negative feelings that your body is having. Yoga can be an art, if it is done correctly. It is easy to learn and something that you will want to continue daily. The results you will see are incredible and can only be improved the more you practice yoga. Men tend to hold their emotions in many different ways; yoga can cure you and treat you in more than one aspect of your life. It is a holistic treatment that treats your mind, body, and spirit.

Men have the same stress and emotions in their minds as women which need to be released. Alternative treatments, such as those listed above, have the power to do this in the most natural way possible. Every year there are more men who are part of these effective alternative treatments for their problems and diseases. The more comfortable society becomes with these alternative treatment methods, the more you will see men taking advantage of their incredible and instantaneous results.

The health of men is very different from that of women, although the same treatments can be used in a different way. The best way to take advantage of these treatments is to find a practitioner to assist you in your search for alternative healing methods. When you start your alternative treatments, you want to make sure that you are using the correct methods for you. These correct methods vary with men and women and, when using the right one, you will find amazing results after the first session.

Alternative treatments for children

There are many diseases that affect children and are difficult to treat. This occurs because it is more difficult to administer conventional treatments to a child, or because the child refuses to take their medication. This is when alternative treatments and medications take place. Children easily accept this type of treatment because they are not associated with traditional medicine; these treatments are something new and exciting for them.

Asthma is a disease that is particularly difficult to treat in children. They do not enjoy using inhalers or any type of treatment that is given. Before you start choosing the treatment for your child, you should remember to keep in mind that these treatments have no scientific endorsement and are not equivalent to conventional medications. These treatments also work only to a certain extent.

Acupuncture

This is a technique in which special needles are inserted into the skin at areas which are key points of the body. Evidence suggests that these needles release endorphins in the brain, which helps reduce pain. Children with asthma who undergo this treatment may find it easier to breathe more calmly and in a relaxed manner.

Hypnosis

This is a treatment that can give children more

self-discipline to continue their medicine on a regular basis.

Massage and relaxation techniques

It has been suggested that stress or anxiety can further constrict the respiratory tract in individuals who suffer from asthma - more so in children than in adults. Massages help reduce stress, assisting the child to breathe easier. You can also learn very good techniques to help control your own breathing patterns. This gives the child the confidence that they can control their own asthma.

There are many other diseases that children have which can be treated with alternative treatments, sometimes used in conjunction with conventional methods. Children with serious illnesses such as cancer or diabetes may need the advantages offered by massages or meditation. Children with diseases that put their lives at risk are prone to retain stress and this can often make their illnesses worse. By using alternative treatments, together with the medicine that your doctor prescribes, you can achieve a very good combination. Sick children need all the help they can get.

As parents, research and diverse opinions of doctors are necessary. Depending on what your child has, you should carefully investigate all the alternative treatments you have in consideration. You must make sure that the treatments will help your child and will not harm them in any way. You will come across treatments such as acupuncture which your child will be reluctant to try. This is the reason why research is something that the child will want to participate in; these treatments are about relaxation and giving your children the confidence that they can control their illness and that they are not alone with it.

Children are more likely to need alternative treatments because they are more reluctant to continue with the medication they prescribed. They are difficult to treat but, if they like the treatment, then everything becomes easier! A good way to get your child excited about your new treatment is to describe it as a gift. Excite them; the more excited they are to try something new, the more they will want to make it part of their daily or weekly routine. As a parent, you should know that your child needs to enjoy what they do, otherwise they will be defeated!

Pay attention to this advice, but make sure that all the ideas you have are reported to your doctor. Alternative treatments can make a big difference in your child's health and attitude!

Alternative medicine for the treatment of cancer

If you have cancer, or know someone who has it, then you know that sometimes the treatment can be as daunting as the disease itself. The effects of chemotherapy can reduce cancer cells, but the side effects include nausea, loss of appetite, and hair loss, to name a few.

It is not surprising that cancer patients seek alternative forms of treatment, and alternative medicine offers some options whose function is to be complementary to the more "modern" forms of treatment. However, there seems to be no middle ground here; while the alternative medicine community is accused of exaggerating the validity of alternative medicine, "conventional" treatment providers tend to underestimate the effects of alternative therapies in people with cancer .

While there is currently no cure for cancer, the NCCAM (National Center for Alternative and Complementary Medicine) has conducted studies demonstrating that acupuncture relieves fatigue, nausea, and painful symptoms associated with colon and breast cancer. It also relieves headaches and neck pain associated with surgery of brain tumors or throat cancer. Ginger is a rich treatment for nausea and vomiting, which are side effects caused by chemotherapy. Hyperbaric oxygen therapy is currently being studied as a relief for cancer of the larynx in patients. This therapy consists of inhaling oxygen with an atmospheric pressure higher than that of sea level. It is being studied as a complement to radiation therapy.

Massage is being used to relieve fatigue caused by any form of cancer.
Another form of alternative therapy used to fight against cancer symptoms is the coupling of pancreatic enzymes with chemotherapy for use in the treatment of pancreatic cancer.
Pancreatic enzymes are proteins secreted by the pancreas that aid in the digestion of food.

There is a difference between complementary

and alternative medicine. Complementary medicine is used in conjunction with conventional medicine, while alternative is used instead of the conventional one. Studies show that better long-term results were obtained with complementary medicine in advanced stages of cancer, while alternative medicine seemed to help in earlier stages of cancer. The study is called MAC, (Complementary Alternative Medicine) and statistics show that 36% of adults at various stages of cancer use both therapies. If you include mega vitamins therapy in this statistic, the numbers almost multiply to 62%. 72% of approximately 500 cancer patients use some form of alternative or complementary therapy for cancer symptoms.

Possibly the most beneficial part of MAC therapy is that patients feel some form of control over their disease; that increases the quality of life and the chances of survival. Bringing relief to pain and giving more hope to cancer patients is a sufficient reason for these foundations to continue receiving grants and continue their studies.

If you are considering MAC therapy, there are some questions you should ask your healthcare provider before starting treatment. One of the most important is, is the treatment covered by the social work and, if so, are there any clauses that you should know about? If the therapy is being sponsored as part of a clinical trial, find out who is sponsoring it, so you will know if the trial is being conducted by an impartial company without marketing credits that can be obtained by the result.

You will also want to ask if the therapy will interfere with any conventional treatment you are receiving at the same time. Normally the answer is no - but you must have all the information before accessing any type of treatment. Ask if there will be any adverse side effects, or if the documented benefits outweigh the risks involved in your case.

Lose weight with alternative medicine

Weight loss is a very important issue which is often discussed on television. If you tune in after 11 PM, you will find several commercials for weight loss pills and dietary supplements, each promising to help you reduce those undesirable extra kilos and end the rolls once and for all. Let's face it, if these pills worked then America would not be at the top of the list of countries with obesity problems.

There are types of alternative medicine which can help you lose weight with great results. While no alternative medicine is a magic solution, practicing these principles can help you become more agile, feel more energetic, and in the end the result (or side effect if you want) is weight loss.

Take yoga as an example; the high impact stretch involved in yoga will help you to feel less stressed and, as a result, not tend to overeat due to depression or anger. Acupuncture uses exact pressure points in the ear that reduce anxiety, detoxifying teas and herbs can help you feel healthier, and the side effect would be to think twice before deciding to "contaminate" yourself again with saturated fat foods. At this point, alternative medicine is wonderful for weight loss.

Most of the alternative medicines for weight loss come in the form of detoxifying teas, energy supplements, and vitamins. The exercise and the dietary plan are the basis for safe, long-term weight loss. There is no magic potion for weight loss; losing weight and maintaining weight requires regular exercise and a change in eating habits.

To prepare for weight loss, here are some detoxifying teas as alternative medicines and some interesting supplements:

Take approximately half a teaspoon of turmeric and ginger, the juice of half a lemon, and boil it all in 2 cups of water. Take it every morning as a detoxifier before you start your diet.

All diets consist of fresh fruits and vegetables; buying a jug is a great way to create a healthy eating habit. Please visit your doctor before starting any type of dietary plan.

Omega three is a good source of nutrients and can be added to any smoothie or juice you are taking.

Visit your neighborhood food store or herbalist, as they can supply you with a variety of alternative teas and nutritional advice. They can recommend a good homeopathic doctor who will evaluate the type of nutrition you need according to your needs.

Bovine and shark cartilage are two dietary supplements that are succeeding in the alternative market. Both have been used for years outside of the United States and Britain, but they are now considered big business in health food stores.

The most popular form of alternative medicine for weight loss is not really medicine itself, but rather behavior modification through hypnosis. Hypnosis does not rely on the power of the will, which is one of the reasons why it is so popular. Hypnosis works by investigating what unconsciously binds the habits of thinking about food and eating, which cause weight gain.

Hypnotists believe that, if the root cause of obesity can be alleviated, the patient will naturally begin to lose weight. It really is a very effective form of alternative medicine and in general they usually cost a lot less than trips to spas or the expensive weight loss pills. Through hypnosis you can let go of fears that prevent you from eating healthily and begin to let positive energy flow through your body, causing you to want to stick to the new way of eating and exercising.

Treatment of neck and back injuries

Many people experience neck and back injuries frequently, which are related to work or just because of incorrect posture or movement. Your neck and back are easy to damage. There are many pills that will prescribe pain relief, but they do not fix the problem and only "cover" the pain for a period of time. More often, alternative treatments are used to cure these injuries.

Injuries to the neck or back can be some of the most painful injuries and you will find yourself weakened for the period of time until the pills take effect. This is not a way of living.

The alternative treatments are very reliable in this field, will fix your injuries, and relieve your pain. These methods are not as in-the-dark as they used to be; they are becoming more and more popular. Here are the alternative treatments that will work better for problems with the neck and back in particular:

- Massage
- Acupuncture

- Meditation

These forms of treatment can be used separately or in combination with one or two. Acupuncture must be the first one to try. If you are not familiar with this technique, let me explain.

Acupuncture is the art of inserting needles in key points of the body. It is believed that these key points release the stress and tension of the body, which is the root of all the pain. Once you get rid of them, you will start to feel better almost instantly. Acupuncture does not involve pain, but relief.

Massages are another way to relieve pain which has become very popular. The massage will release the tension of your muscles and will balance your body. It is something that will need to be used several times in a month to be effective. Depending on the severity of the injury, it should be more frequent than this. Massage can almost always help; it may even be a good idea to combine it with acupuncture.

Meditation is a very strong healing method that is used as an alternative treatment. It is a method that heals the soul as well as the mind.

This may sound like it will not do anything to cure the injuries to your neck and back, but assuming this would be wrong. The condition of your mind and soul are as important as your physical condition and meditation is an art; it requires a lot of self-discipline and concentration.

It can work if you put the effort into making it work. With regard to injuries, it is best to combine meditation with acupuncture or massage. Meditation is something that you will want to start practicing daily. It can help you with not only injuries, but with other diseases you may have.

Alternative treatments are very good for healing injuries; remember that it may be better to combine one or two of these treatments to achieve the maximum effect. You can also combine conventional medical treatments with one of these great alternative treatments. Your objective is the maximum benefit; it will be better for you to consult with an alternative medicine doctor before starting any of these treatments. You can receive good advice, learn more about these alternative methods, and feel more confident when using them. Alternative treatments can make a difference and treat injuries with great healing power.

Five tips for gathering mind and spirit

What is your passion? What is it that brings together your body, mind, and spirit? Whether it's daily meditation or prayer, a rigid diet system, or just a good book, the result of being able to combine these three aspects of yourself can bring the balance that most people want to have in their lives.

Although we talk a lot about balance, most people leave out the concept of the soul - mostly because it is not very well understood by Westerners. I suppose that what makes your soul move is also what causes you to feel the kind of energy that can only be described as passion.

That does not mean sexual passion, but spiritual passion. The best example I know of, for me at least, is listening to the gospel music of Bautista del Sur. This kind of music uplifts me and reminds me that there is a world much bigger than my own out there, so I ask again, what are you passionate about? Here are five tips that help you decide:

Set goals for the future

Future goals are supposed to inspire passion; are yours worthy of your body, mind, and spirit?

Please do not tell me it has to do with money, which is good if that is what matters to you, but it should be the process of pursuing these goals that inspires passion. What makes the end goal so much sweeter is the journey to achieve it. Set a goal to explore three new forms of spirituality this season, for example.

Remember your achievements

One of the best ways to nourish your body, mind, and spirit is to remember how much good you do and not to get discouraged by every little mistake.

The quickest way to crush your soul is to constantly tell yourself that you are useless, that you ruin everything. Your soul and mind will eventually believe it and your body will get sick.

Create Scenes of Joy

This is a form of meditation in which you practice taking your mind to a happy and safe place that it creates or plans to visit someday. When stress attacks your mind, go to your safe place for a minute. (Yes, this advice is parodied in movies all the time, but it does work.)

Wait for something plan a getaway

Nothing seems to nourish the body, mind, and spirit more than to physically go and find a new place to explore, even for a weekend. Plan a weekend trip and go to the mountains or the beach, in whatever direction your heart takes you. Now here is the best part -go alone. When was the last time you spent some time outside without anyone other than yourself? This can be very relaxing and you do not have to worry about entertaining anyone other than you.

Practice affirmations, find a relief for stress, and practice it

We have already briefly discussed this in point

two, but make three affirmations and say them out loud in front of the mirror every day. This has been proven to work! If you say something about yourself enough times, it will come true. It seems so easy for people to believe when it comes to negative things about ourselves, so why is it so hard to believe that it will work the other way too?

Here are three simple statements for you to start:

"I'm always safe and secure."
"The universe provides me with everything I need." "My income is increasing."

Chapter 13 – Final Words

The Chinese have long been masters of caring for and restoring the body naturally. The Chinese were convinced that the diseases came from physical inactivity and therefore practiced kung fu, which were exercises that combined stretching and correct breathing to preserve the organic functions.

Long before the Christian era there were already several schools in China where children and adults practiced kung fu. With this comment we mean that this town traditionally gave much importance to the care of the body in a natural way.

In the West, the techniques of traditional Chinese medicine such as acupuncture, acupressure, tai chi gymnastics, and others, have been recognized and applied only in recent decades.

The truth is that, from childhood, we should learn the main preventive measures to care for and maintain the health of the spine.

As well as gymnastics or sports classes, there should be regular courses on this important subject. In addition, gymnastics (which tends to strive towards achieving vigorous minds and bodies) should focus more on the improvement of the general state of health.

On the contrary, many problems in the column begin to creep in from childhood. There are those who adopt the stoop pose because they are shy. There are others who grow up suddenly, especially those who reach heights above six feet, who find it difficult to correctly handle their posture and begin to deflect their spine. Or there are sports fans, some of them having quite abrupt and frequent collisions which produce unsurprising injuries.

The truth is that, since childhood, you have to acquire that culture of care for the body and its functions under the protection and education of the elderly. When you become an adult, the responsibility changes hands.

Eating healthily, taking care of controlling negative emotions, performing low-impact physical activities, and adhering to activities that distract the mind are some of the things that an adult should keep under strict control. If the adult has small children who still depend on their responsibility, they should strive to teach those essential care routines that ensure a good quality of life – children learn best through following an example.

Throughout this book, we wanted to be practical and abound in knowledge that will serve life. The Second Part is entirely dedicated to learning and adopting habits that improve the health of the spine and the entire area of the back, as well as helping to prevent future problems.

We believe that if someone listens to us and a rigorous plan is established with all the recommendations, very soon they will feel better and will be able to enjoy every moment of their existence. Of course, you will have to be persistent.

You can also try the huge amount of body techniques designed to relieve back pain as performed by physiotherapists, osteopaths, or chiropractors. You have to ensure you place yourself in the hands of professionals of proven ability in the techniques they practice, who take into account the patient in the physical as well as the emotional sense.

Finally, we leave our readers some practical tips that they should not forget every day:

- Avoid bad postures: stand and walk correctly, sit properly, and adopt the best position to sleep.
- Do not lift heavy objects.
- Relieve tension.
- Leave aside any situation that involves continuous stress.
- Eat in a healthy, nutritious, and balanced way.
- Control body weight.
- No smoking.
- Relieve back pain with cold and hot packs.

- Avoid medication as much as possible, which may cause side effects.

- Perform physical activity on a regular basis, which contains stretching and breathing exercises.

- Adhere to alternative medicines that may be beneficial.

- Be happy! Enjoy all the good the comes with being alive.

We wish all our readers good luck and that they can overcome their back-related ailments, naturally improve their organic and neuromuscular capacities, and that they find a way to express their emotions through creative activities that allow them to see life in its most positive phase.

Thank you very much for trusting in our words. Congratulations!

- Erika Sanders

Glossary

Acupuncture. Therapeutic resource of traditional Chinese medicine that uses very fine needles applied to the meridian of the pain area.

Arachondritis. Inflammation of the arachnoid lining of the brain and spinal cord, which causes chronic pain mainly in the lower back and lower limbs.

Arthritis. Inflammation of the joints.

Arthrosis. Pathological alteration of the joints, which is of a degenerative nature (it shows certain changes) although not inflammatory.

Swiss ball or ball (in English, swiss ball). Elastic sphere widely used in therapeutic exercises. It serves to make exercises and also to relax the body.

Dorsal kyphosis. Curvature of the spine in the area of the dorsal vertebrae that is convex backwards.

Coccigodynia. Pain in the coccyx or sweet bone.

Spine. Also called spine. Joint of articulated bones that extends from the base of the skull to the birth of the lower limbs, where it is joined to the hip by means of the iliac sacral joints. It results in the support of the body as well as the protection of the spinal cord.

Spinal dislocation. Vertebra or misaligned vertebrae.

Pain. Alarm sign and annoying sensation of a part of the body, which can range from mild to acute. It is a fundamental part of the body's communication with the brain. Pain is a subjective sensation, because in the same symptom, not all people feel it with the same intensity.

Scoliosis. Abnormal curvature in the spine.

Endorphins. Natural substances created by the body that function as neurotransmitters. They are produced by the pituitary gland and the hypothalamus, after exercise, excitement, joy, some foods. They provoke an analgesic effect and provide a feeling of well-being.

Back. (from the Latin, spathula). Back of the

human body, which goes from the shoulders to the waist.

Isthmic spondylolisthesis. Herniated disc.

Spinal stenosis. Narrowing of the spinal canal due to the growth of bones or tissues.

Physiotherapy. (from Greek, physis, nature, and therapeia, treatment). Specialty of medicine that for the prevention, the healing and the recovery, as much resorts to natural elements as to mechanical actions.

Fracture. Bone break or break.

Fracture-dislocation. Break or break combination with vertebral misalignment.

Cervical lordosis. Curvature of the spine in the area of the cervical vertebrae that is concave backwards.

Lumbar lordosis. Curvature of the spine in the area of the lumbar vertebrae that is concave backwards.

Lumbago (from the Latin, lumbago). Pain located in the back.

Spinal cord. Part of the cerebrospinal system contained in the spinal canal.

Osteopathy. Holistic alternative medicine to restore body balance, relieve pain and restore organic functions. It uses techniques such as energy and stretching.

Articular osteopathy. Focus your work to relieve pain and restore organic functions in the spine.

Pilates. Gymnastic method designed by Joseph Pilates, ideal to correct incorrect body postures. Works muscle strength and endurance.

Prana. For certain spiritual conceptions, subtle vital energy.

Chiropractic. Physical therapy techniques that focus on the manipulation of the spine for its alignment and its relationship with the central nervous system. Consider that the body has the ability to heal and regulate itself.

Vertebral subluxation. A vertebra moves or moves out of alignment with respect to one or both of the adjacent vertebrae, causing pressure on the nerve.

Vertebra (from the Latin, vertebra). Each of the small bones or ossicles that make up the spine or spine. The vertebrae as a whole are traversed by the spinal cord.

Yoga (from the Sanskrit yuj, union). Method or system designed to achieve mental, physical and spiritual development.

contained herein.

The information in this book may not be compatible with conventional medicine or the opinions of some doctors. However, it is well documented and supported by many doctors, scientists, and health professionals. Before starting any practice related to health, diet, or exercise, it is highly recommended that you consult your doctor.

CPSIA information can be obtained
at www.ICGtesting.com
Printed in the USA
BVHW040947080221
599619BV00006B/123